Senses

Written by Hazel Songhurst

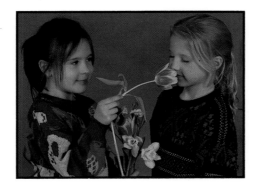

Wayland

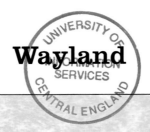

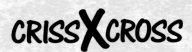

CRISS**X**CROSS

Picture acknowledgements

The publishers would like to thank the following for allowing their photographs to be reproduced in this book. Bruce Coleman Ltd. 8 (Jane Burton), 9 (above/ P. Carr), 19 (Kim Taylor), 22 (above/Jane Burton), 22 (below/Kim Taylor), 23 (Jane Burton), 26 (below/John Visser), 28 (Kim Taylor), 29 (above/Jeff Foott Productions), 29 (below/CB and DW Frith); Context Picture Library 12 (below/ Tizzie Knowles); Reflections (all Jennie Woodcock) 5 (below), 6 (below), 7 (above), 7 (below), 15 (above), 20 (above), 26 (above); Eye Ubiquitous 14 (below/Peter Palmer), 16 (PS), 17 (Yiorgos Nikiteas); Tony Stone Worldwide 5 (above/Arthur Tilley), 6 (above), 10, 11 (above/George Dore), 13 (Lisa Valder), 14 (above/Hans Reinhard), 21, 24 (Jo Browne/Mick Smee), 25 (below/Peter Comez), 27 (Ron Sutherland); ZEFA *cover*, 4, 9 (below), 11 (below), 15, 18 (above), 18 (below), 20 (below), 25 (above/both).

First published in 1993 by
Wayland (Publishers) Ltd
61 Western Road, Hove
East Sussex BN3 1JD, England

© Copyright 1993 Wayland (Publishers) Ltd

Editor: Francesca Motisi
Designer: Jean Wheeler

Consultant: Alison Watkins is an experienced teacher with a special interest in language and reading. She has been a class teacher and the special needs coordinator for a school in Hackney. Alison wrote the notes for parents and teachers and provided the topic web.

British Library Cataloguing in Publication Data
Songhurst, Hazel.
Senses. – (Criss Cross)
I. Title II. Series
612.8

ISBN 0-7502-0764-7

Typeset by DJS Fotoset Ltd, Brighton, Sussex
Printed and bound in Italy by L.E.G.O. S.p.A., Vicenza

Contents

Words that appear in **bold** in the text are explained in the glossary on page 32.

Collecting information

You have five senses – sight, hearing, smell, taste and touch. They are hard at work all the time collecting **information** about the world around you.

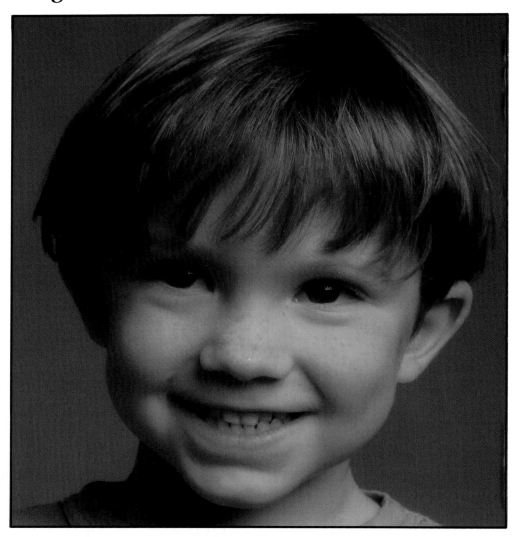

The parts of your body which collect information are called sense organs. They are your eyes, skin, tongue, nose, ears and inner ear.

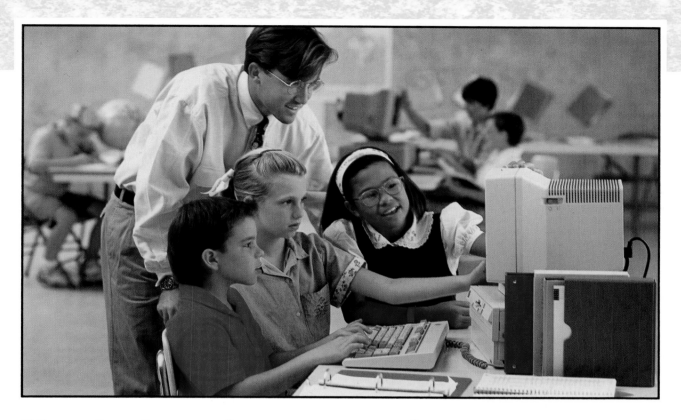

Your **brain** receives messages from your senses and works out what they mean. What senses are these children using?

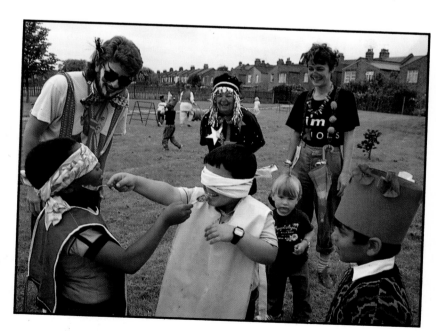

These children are playing a game wearing blindfolds. Their sense of sight has been taken away from them.

Sight

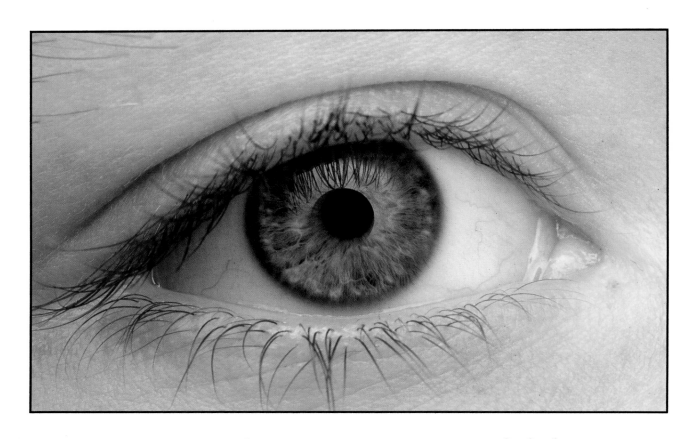

Your eyes give you your sense of sight.
You can see by using your eyes.

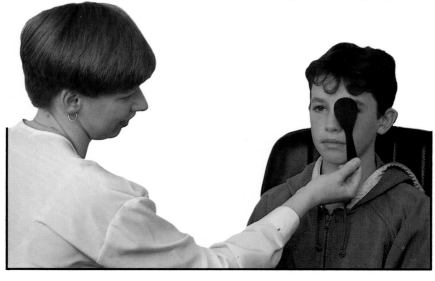

This boy is having
his eyes tested by
an **optician**.

6

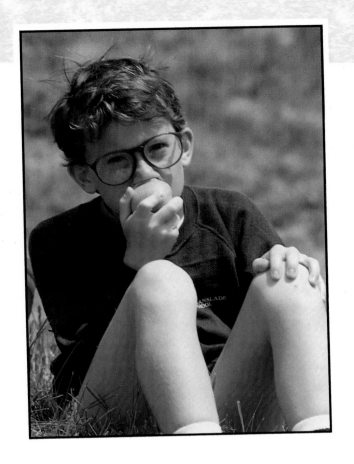

People who cannot see very well wear glasses to help them see more clearly.

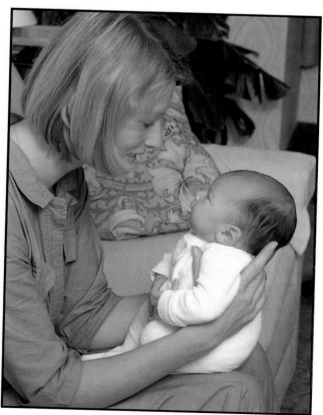

When babies are born their eyes do not **focus** properly at first. This mother is holding her baby close to her face so that it can see her more easily.

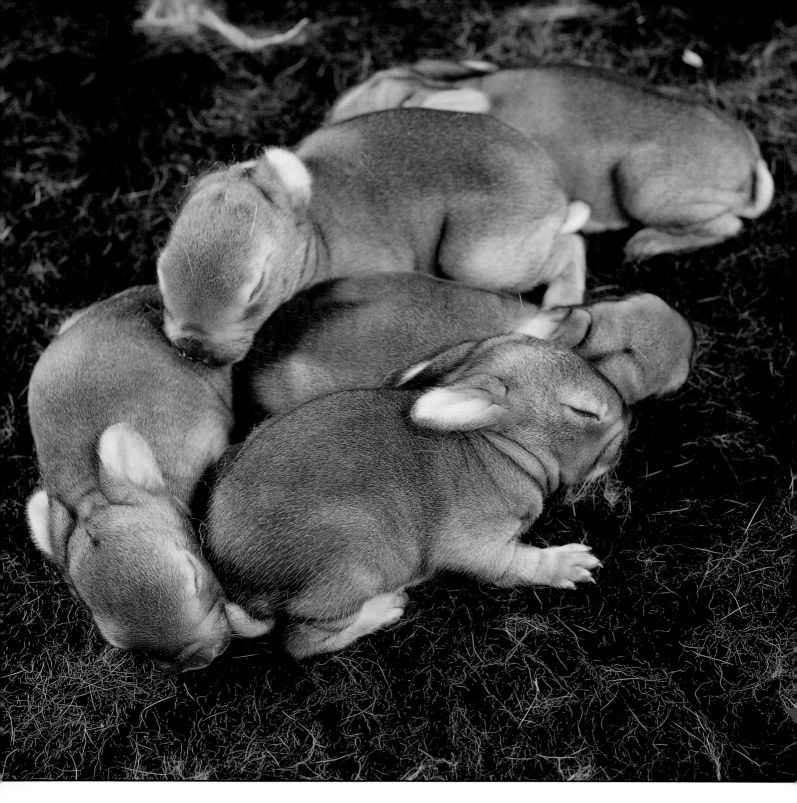

Many baby animals are **blind** when they are first born. These baby rabbits have their eyes tightly closed but they will soon open.

Hunting animals have very good eyesight. This owl uses its big eyes to see the mice and other small animals it hunts.
What other hunting animals do you know?

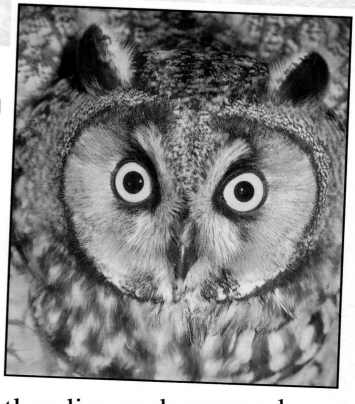

Moles are nearly blind. Their sense of sight is not important to them because they live underground.

This bushbaby has big eyes to help it see in the dark. Bushbabies usually sleep during the day and move around at night.

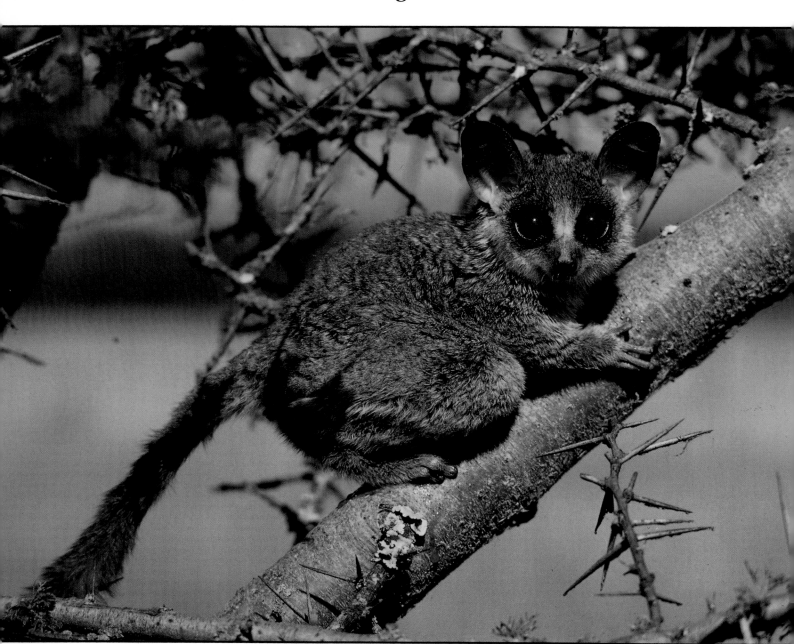

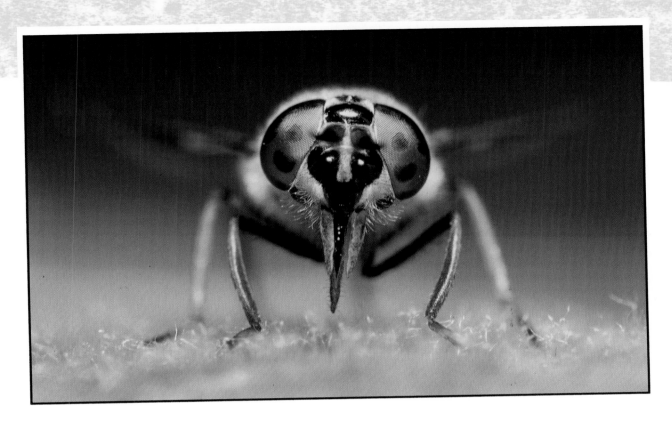

This insect's eye is made up of hundreds of tiny **lenses**. Insects have **fuzzy** eyesight but they can see the smallest movement straight away.

Snails' eyes are on stalks high above their bodies.

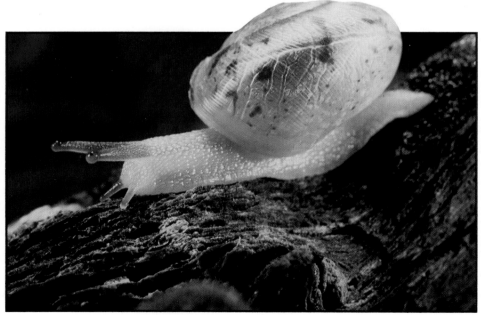

Hearing

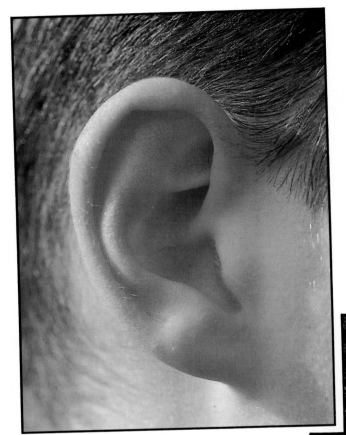

The outside part of your ears collect sound and guide it into the small hole that leads to the inside part of your ears. It is the inside part of your ears that gives you your sense of hearing.

Your hearing lets you hear warning sounds, and sounds such as music, that make you happy. But most important, it lets you hear other people talking.

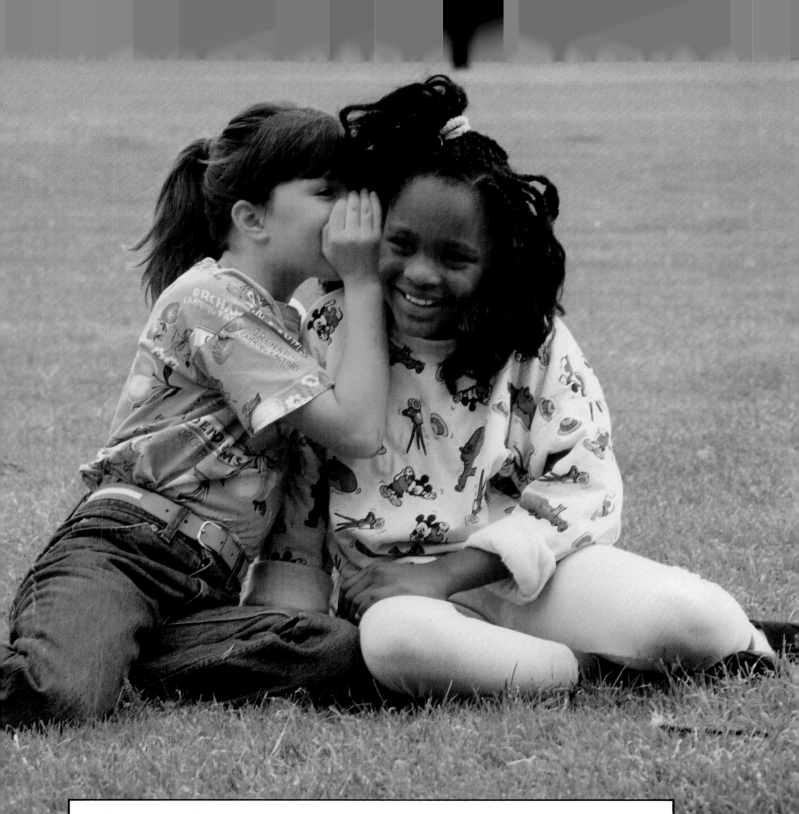

We can hear high sounds, low sounds, loud sounds and soft, whispering sounds.

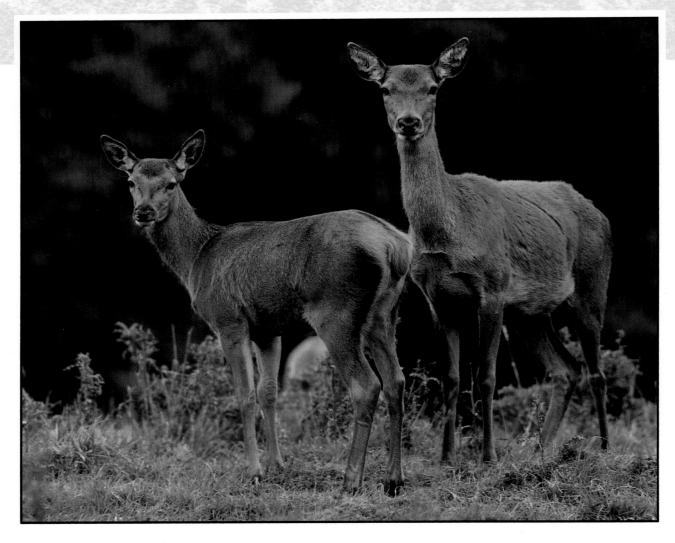

Most animals can hear much better than people. Deers have large ears. They can turn them to pick up sounds from all around.

Birds have no outer ears. Their feathers cover small ear-holes on either side of their heads.

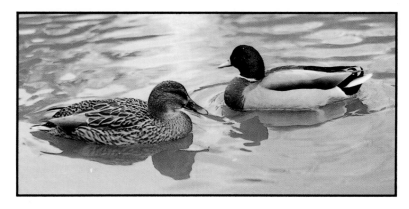

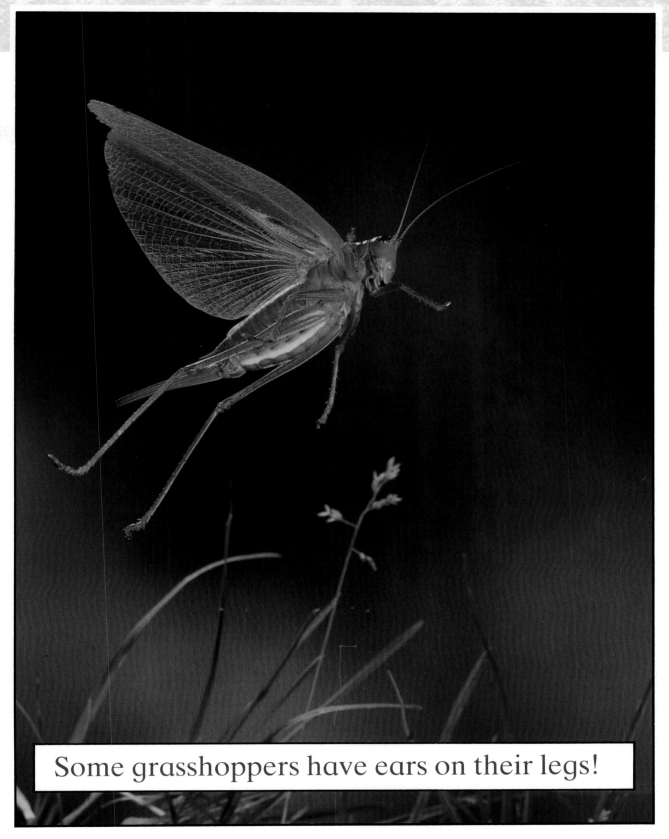

Some grasshoppers have ears on their legs!

Smell

Your nose gives you your sense of smell. You can smell by breathing in through your nose.

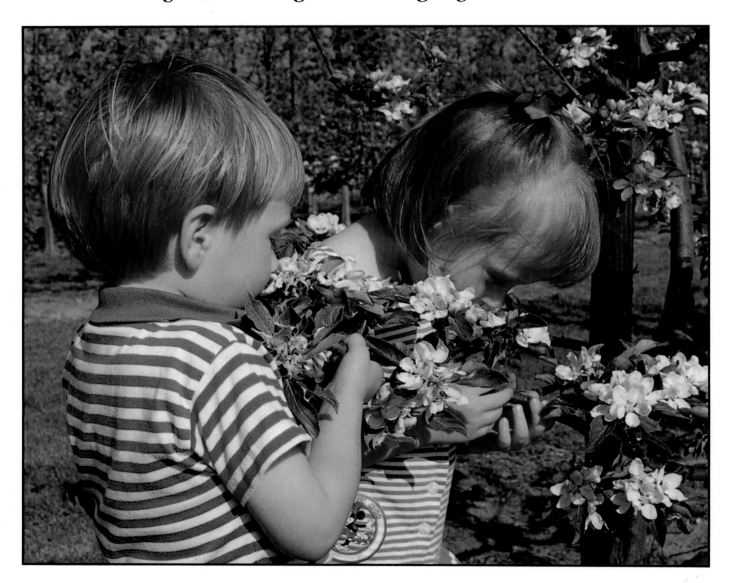

We like nice smells, such as the **scent** of flowers, or delicious food. Nasty smells, such as smoke or bad food, warn us to keep away.

16

When you have a cold you can lose your sense of smell for a while.

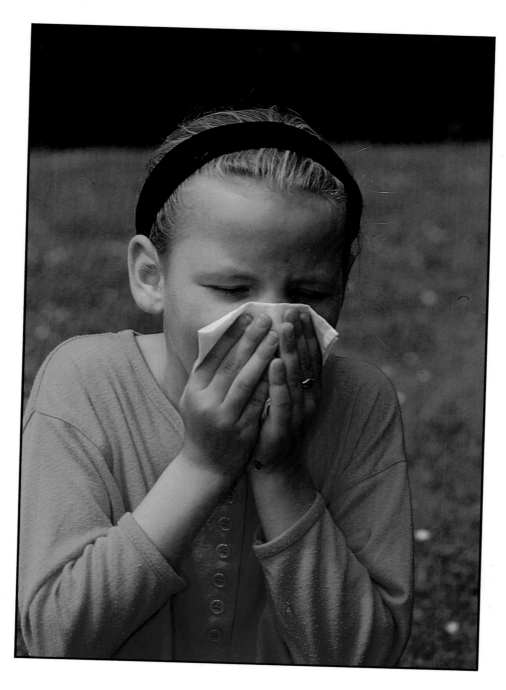

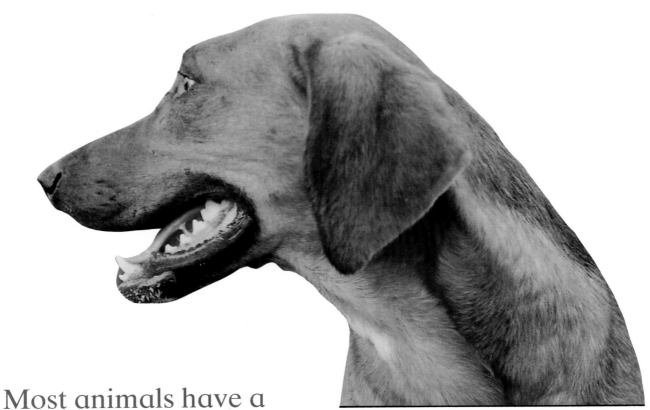

Most animals have a much stronger sense of smell than people. Dogs have a very good sense of smell.

Did you know fish have a good sense of smell? Salmon use their sense of smell to find their way back to the place where they were born.

18

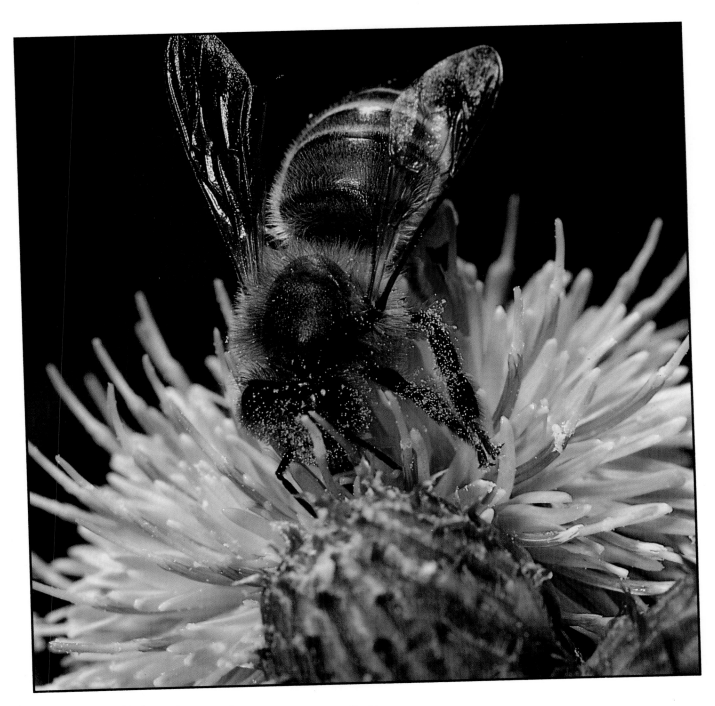

The lovely scent of flowers attracts bees and other flying insects.

Taste

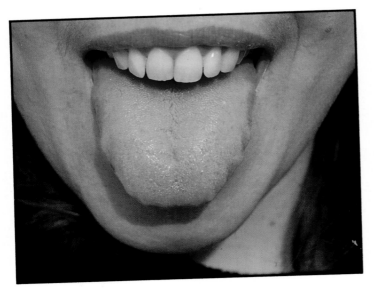

All over your tongue are tiny bumps called taste-buds. They tell you the different tastes of food and drink.

Different parts of your tongue are used for different tastes. You can taste sweet and salty tastes with the tip, and sour and bitter tastes at the sides and back. Which is your favourite kind of taste?

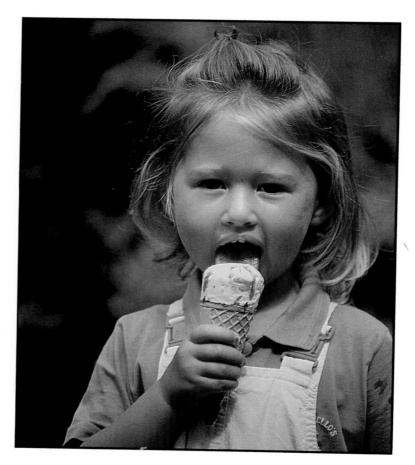

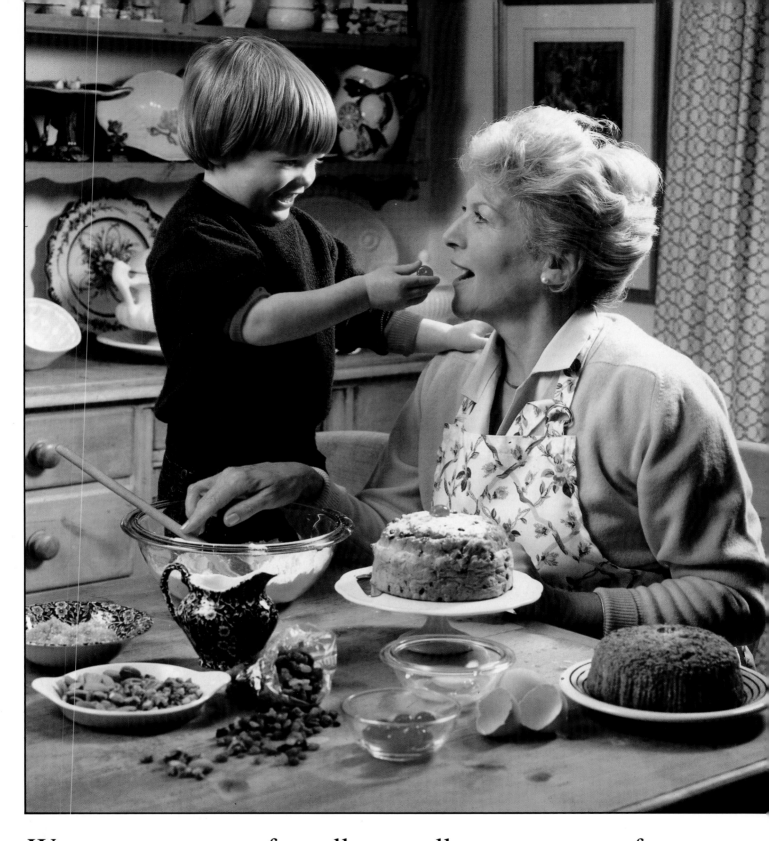

We use our sense of smell, as well as our sense of taste, to help us recognize flavours.

Snakes have long forked tongues that can feel and smell, as well as taste things. What other animals with forked tongues do you know?

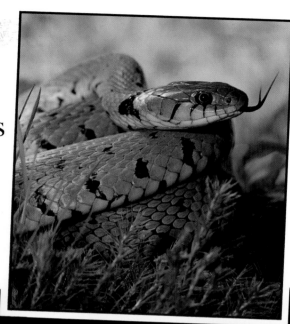

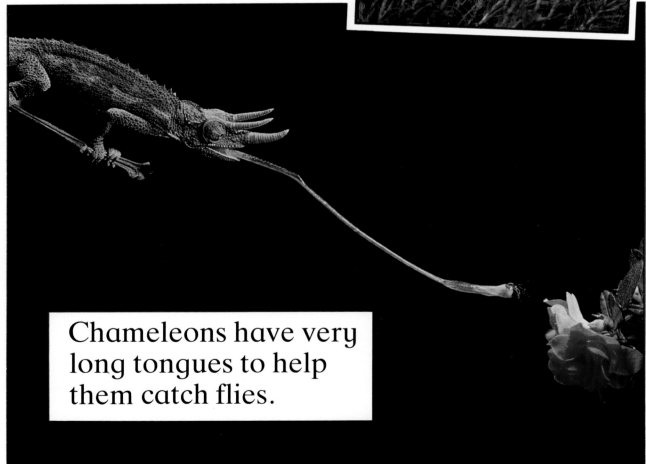

Chameleons have very long tongues to help them catch flies.

A kiss can make you feel much better!

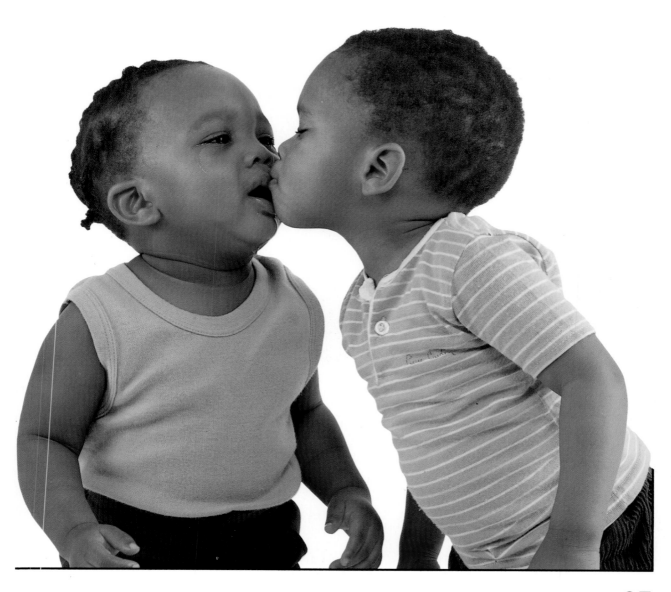

Supersenses

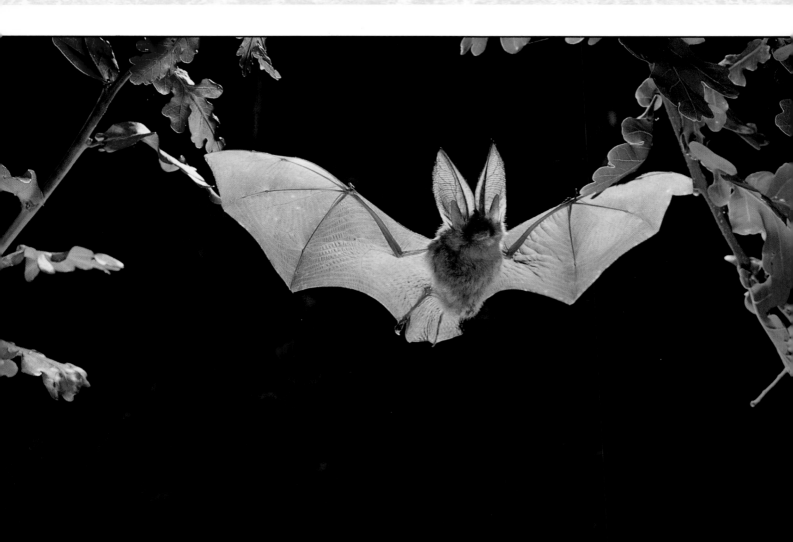

Many animals have far better senses than people. We call them supersenses. When a bat hunts it sends out very high-pitched sounds that hit flying insects and make echoes. The echoes bounce back to the bat and it knows exactly where to find its **prey**.

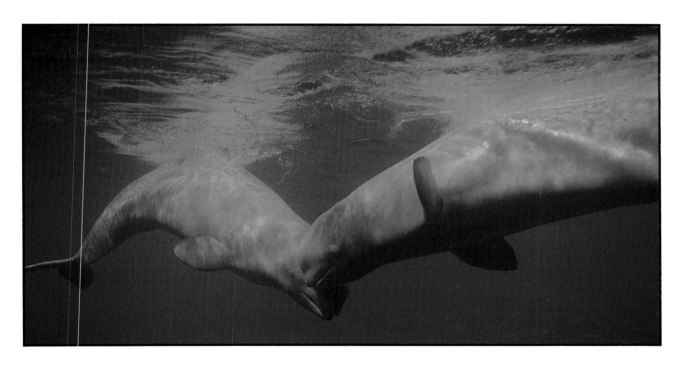

Sound travels faster through water than through air. Whales, dolphins and porpoises also use echoes to help them find food.

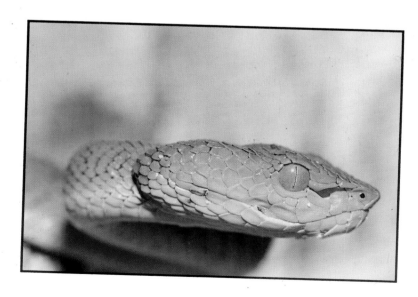

Some snakes have a special place between their eyes and nostrils that can feel when prey is nearby.

Notes for parents and teachers

Science
- Investigate how sound travels by playing a variety of instruments and feeling for the vibrations.
- Hearing sounds from a distance. Discover which sounds travel furthest. Try different children's voices. Are they easy to identify?
- Distinguish between fair and unfair tests eg tests for:– keen/sharp hearing, using one ear or two, touch tests and distribution of touch receptors over the body, listening and identifying sounds.

English
- Make your name or a word out of textured paper or material, so the letters can be felt. Which are the easiest/hardest to feel? Is this because of the texture used, or the length of the name?
- Develop children's listening skills by asking them to listen to sounds around them. They should then write down or draw any sounds they heard. Also use tapes of familiar sounds for the children to identify.

Art
- Recognize different kinds of art and different artists. Look at and talk about examples of work from artists who painted using their feet or mouth.
- Make collections, for example of pebbles, and arrange in order of colour, or put into sets according to shape or texture.

Drama
- Arrange a visit to a local optician and then change your home corner into one. The children can make charts to test someone's eyes. They can also experiment with optical illusions.
- Sit in a circle with a blind-folded person sitting in the middle guarding a bunch of keys. Who can steal the keys from the guard?

History
- Find out about Louis Braille, the Frenchman who discovered a way to make writing which people with visual disabilities can 'read' by touching.
- Also find out about Sir Edward Henry who was the Commissioner of the London Police from 1903-1919. He worked out a way of catching criminals by discovering that no two people have the same pattern of prints on their fingertips.

Geography
- Go on an exploratory walk to investigate how we use our senses to explore our environment.

D.T.
- Design devices or aids to help people who have a visual or hearing disability, eg a buzzer that will light up. Also think about your own home or school and how people with no sight would be able to move around.

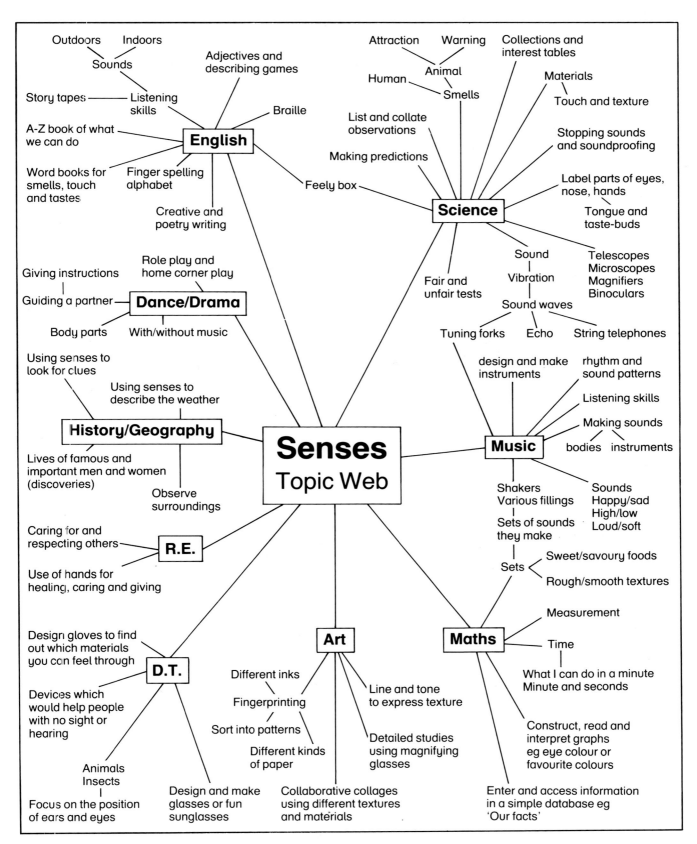

Senses
Topic Web

English
- Outdoors
- Indoors
- Sounds
- Story tapes — Listening skills
- A-Z book of what we can do
- Word books for smells, touch and tastes
- Finger spelling alphabet
- Adjectives and describing games
- Braille
- Creative and poetry writing

Dance/Drama
- Giving instructions
- Guiding a partner
- Body parts
- Role play and home corner play
- With/without music

History/Geography
- Using senses to look for clues
- Using senses to describe the weather
- Lives of famous and important men and women (discoveries)
- Observe surroundings

R.E.
- Caring for and respecting others
- Use of hands for healing, caring and giving

D.T.
- Design gloves to find out which materials you can feel through
- Devices which would help people with no sight or hearing
- Animals Insects
- Focus on the position of ears and eyes

Art
- Different inks
- Fingerprinting
- Sort into patterns
- Different kinds of paper
- Line and tone to express texture
- Detailed studies using magnifying glasses
- Design and make glasses or fun sunglasses
- Collaborative collages using different textures and materials

Science
- Attraction
- Warning
- Human
- Animal
- Smells
- Collections and interest tables
- Materials
- Touch and texture
- List and collate observations
- Making predictions
- Feely box
- Stopping sounds and soundproofing
- Label parts of eyes, nose, hands
- Tongue and taste-buds
- Fair and unfair tests
- Sound
- Vibration
- Sound waves
- Telescopes Microscopes Magnifiers Binoculars
- Tuning forks
- Echo
- String telephones

Music
- design and make instruments
- rhythm and sound patterns
- Listening skills
- Making sounds
- bodies   instruments
- Shakers Various fillings
- Sets of sounds they make
- Sets
- Sounds Happy/sad High/low Loud/soft
- Sweet/savoury foods
- Rough/smooth textures

Maths
- Measurement
- Time
- What I can do in a minute Minute and seconds
- Construct, read and interpret graphs eg eye colour or favourite colours
- Enter and access information in a simple database eg 'Our facts'

31

Index

Glossary

Blind   A blind person or animal cannot see.

Braille   Special printing (invented by Louis Braille) for people who cannot see. The letters are made with raised dots and are read by feeling them with the fingertips.

Brain   Your brain is inside your skull. It controls your body.

Focus   When your eyes focus they see something clearly.

Fuzzy   Eyesight that is fuzzy is not clear, but is blurred.

Information   Something you need to know about e.g. facts, news, etc.

Lenses   The lens in your eye is the part that focuses light and makes you see clearly. Some insects's eyes have many lenses.

Optician   An optician is a person who tests your eyes and sells glasses and contact lenses.

Prey   The animals hunted by other animals as food are called prey.

Receptors   Parts of your body that receive special messages from your senses.

Scent   The scent of something is its particular smell.